LIVING & THRIVING WITH HEAD & NECK CANCER

Danko Martincic, MD

Richard O. Wein, MD, FACS

Heather Gabbert, MS, RD, LD

Kathy Beach, RN

Christopher M. Lee, MD

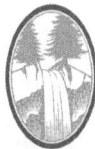

**PROVENIR
PUBLISHING**
Spokane, Washington

Living & Thriving With Head & Neck Cancer

The authors, editors, and publisher have made every effort to provide accurate information. However, they are not responsible for errors, omissions, or for any outcomes related to the use of contents of this book and take no responsibility for the use of the products and procedures described. Treatments and side effects described in this book may not be applicable to all people; likewise, some people may require a different treatment than described herein due to individual circumstances. Drugs and medical devices are discussed, but may have limited availability controlled by the Food and Drug Administration (FDA) for use only in a research study or clinical trial. Research, clinical practice, and government relations often change the accepted standard in the field. When consideration is being given to use of any drug in a clinical setting, the health care provider or reader is responsible for determining the optimal treatment for an individual patient and is responsible for reviewing the most up-to-date recommendations on dose, precautions, and contra indications, and determining the appropriate usage for the product. This is especially important in the case of drugs that are new or seldom used.

Published by Provenir Publishing, LLC, P. O. Box 211, Greenacres, WA 99016-0211

Production Credits

Editors: Christopher Lee and Micah Harman

Production Director: Amy Hanson

Art Director and Illustration: Micah Harman

Cover Photo: Micah Harman

Printing History: June 2012, First Edition.

This book is dedicated to all of our inspirational and insightful patients who are resolved to conquer cancer.

CONTENTS

If you are holding this book in your hand, it is likely that you, a close family member, or close friend has been diagnosed with a cancer of the nose, sinuses, neck, mouth, or throat. In most cases, this diagnosis is a shock and came from "out of the blue." You probably have 1000 questions floating around in your head; like how this diagnosis will be treated, how you will feel, how this will affect your family and your work, and what should you do next. Any cancer diagnosis has an impact on many facets of life. This is a fact. The goal of this book is to provide you with knowledge about your diagnosis and to assist in clarifying procedures, alleviate fears, and optimize your treatment. Our hope is that this is written in such a way that it assists in also alleviating symptoms as well as answering questions that commonly come up with a cancer diagnosis. We also have included a section on practical nutritional techniques that can add to your ability to heal, improve your immune health, and optimize your energy and overall health.

Cancers of the head and neck affect patients in a wide variety of ways and perhaps more than in any other group of patients require a team of physicians and health care providers to assist on this path of treatment.

The goal of this book is to compile experience and expertise in a way that can be easily interpreted and provide rapid assistance in answering questions and provide guidance to you in your cancer journey.

PART ONE

What Is Cancer?

What is cancer? Cancer by definition is an uncontrolled growth of cells which were once normal within the body, and are now growing in an uncontrolled way and destroying the function of surrounding normal cells. Cancer can involve a single organ of the body or in some circumstances can spread through the bloodstream to other organs (metastasize). Cells normally divide through a normal predictable process and cancer is a condition where the cells fail to follow their normal process due to damage to the DNA. DNA is the substance within every cell that directs its activities and processes. In normal circumstances, your body is continually repairing DNA damage due to the environment, but in cancer cells the damaged DNA is not repaired. In some people, they develop inherited damaged DNA which accounts for inherited cancers. More often, the DNA damage occurs due to exposure to something in the environment; for example, environmental carcinogens in pesticides, cigarette use, or alcohol use.

Different types of cancer can behave differently; for example, cancers of the tonsil or tongue can behave very differently from a cancer of the lung. They grow at different rates and respond to different types of treatment. This is why patients with cancer need treatment specifically directed at their cancer type and with modern drugs and technology. Due to years of research, modern cancer therapy is tailored to each person's individual situation and their overall health.

Approximately 45,000 patients are diagnosed each year in the United States with nose, sinus, mouth, and throat cancer. These cancers which are termed "head and neck cancers" refer to abnormal cells that arise from and grow in different organs of the body all found above the shoulders (except for the brain and spinal cord). In addition, the exact area within the head and neck that these tumors arise from can lead to the cancers having different characteristics; for example, cancer of the tongue is very different from a cancer of the voice box, and they are each treated very differently. The cells of the tongue also look different under the microscope from the cells of the voice box (larynx).

The main organs in the head and neck area from which tumors can arise are termed the pharynx (which includes the nasopharynx, hypopharynx, and oropharynx) as well as the nasal sinuses (ethmoid, sphenoid, maxillary), oral cavity (tongue, cheeks, floor of mouth and palate), and larynx.

PART TWO

How Do I Know If I Have Cancer?

MAIN SYMPTOMS OF HEAD AND NECK CANCER

The symptoms experienced by people when they are diagnosed with head and neck cancer can vary depending upon the site of the cancer origin. In truth, you may have experienced very different symptoms from your head and neck cancer diagnosis than someone else who has been diagnosed with a cancer in the very same organ.

THE MOST COMMON SYMPTOMS THAT PEOPLE EXPERIENCE ARE:

- A lump or sore that does not heal
- A new lump or mass in the neck
- Difficulty with jaw or tongue motion
- Hoarseness of the voice
- Changes in how the teeth feel or dentures fit
- Persistent swollen glands or lymph nodes in the neck
- Loss of smell
- Nasal discharge
- Coughing up blood
- Persistent nasal congestion
- Mouth or jaw pain
- New growing white or red patches on the inside lining of the mouth

Of course, if someone has any of these new symptoms, they should consult with their physician immediately for an exam.

During an examination by your doctor, they may examine the oral and nasal cavities as well as the neck, throat, and tongue using a small mirror or light as well as potentially using a small camera on the end of a tube which can look inside of your nose and down behind your tongue at the larynx and examine the vocal cord motion. Common tests that are also ordered,

fig. 2.1

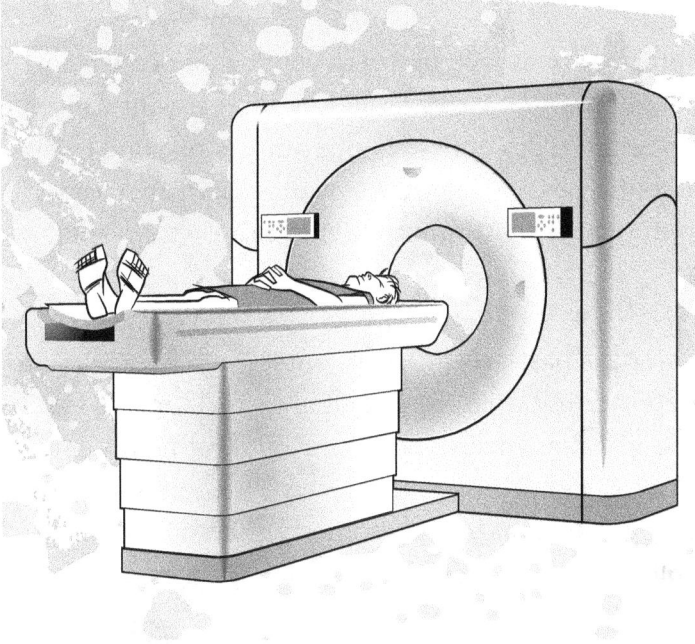

CT scans allow your doctors to map out the extent of the cancer spread.

if there is a suspicion of cancer, are blood tests as well as imaging studies [such as x-rays, CT (or CAT) scans, magnetic resonance imaging (MRI), or also PET scans].

Depending upon their examination and the results of the imaging studies, a biopsy may be required. A biopsy is simply a procedure which involves removing a small amount of cells or tissues (biopsy specimen) in the affected area so that they can be examined under a microscope by a physician who specializes in tissue identification (Pathologist). A Pathologist will often be able to determine how aggressive they appear under a microscope and the specific type of cellularity involved (where the tumor has originated from). This

NURSE'S NOTE:

Pathologists can use special tests to determine the origin and aggressiveness of cancer

NURSE'S NOTE:

Smoking is a tough habit to quit. Your nurse can direct you to helpful resources that can aid in success.

information is very useful to your cancer care team in determining the optimal way to treat your cancer. Different types of tissues and cancers respond to different types of chemotherapy drugs and are treated optimally by customized therapies.

RISK FACTORS FOR HEAD AND NECK CANCER

Over the past decades, a lot of research has gone into determining what the potential risk factors are for these malignancies so that preventative treatments can be used. Through this research, scientists have recognized that patient or lifestyle factors can play a role in the risk of developing a malignancy.

RISK FACTORS FOR HEAD AND NECK CANCER INCLUDE:

- *Age* (these cancers occur most often in patients who are over the age of 50). Of course, younger people can also develop cancer in the head and neck area, although this is much less common statistically.
- *Gender* (men are 3 to 4 times more likely than women to get head and neck cancer (however, this is changing as women are now increasing their use of tobacco products)
- *Race* (cancer of the lip occurs predominantly in Caucasian males)
- *Nasopharynx cancers* are endemic to parts of China and in Chinese Americans born in the United States
- *Specific molecular markers* have also been determined to play a role in the aggressiveness and development of cancers

such as p53 gene mutations and over expression of the Epidermal Growth Factor Receptor (abbreviated EGFR, this is a known target on the surface of cancer cells which are effected by new biotherapies such as the drug Erbitux)

- *Tobacco use*
- *Alcohol use*
- *Dietary factors*
- *Gastric Reflux*
- *Environmental and occupational exposures to chemicals* at the workplace
- *Sun exposure*
- *Other medical conditions*
- *Human Papilloma Virus Exposure (HPV).* Over the last decade, scientists have found that many head and neck cancers are started by a viral exposure such as HPV (human papilloma virus). For example, recent studies have shown that approximately 60% of the cancers of the oropharynx (tonsils, throat, and base of tongue) currently are due to HPV infections.

YOUR CANCER TEAM AND TOOLS FOR TREATMENT

Because of the complexities of cancer therapy and the uniqueness of each individual and their situation, the optimal way to treat head and neck cancer is by using a team approach (otherwise known as a "Multidisciplinary Approach"). During the phase of time where

NURSE'S NOTE:

Seeing multiple care specialists can be tiring. Keeping these appointments is important to assure every aspect of treatment is addressed.

someone has been newly diagnosed and is undergoing the initial tests and procedures to determine their type of cancer and extensiveness, patients are usually referred to a team of specialists.

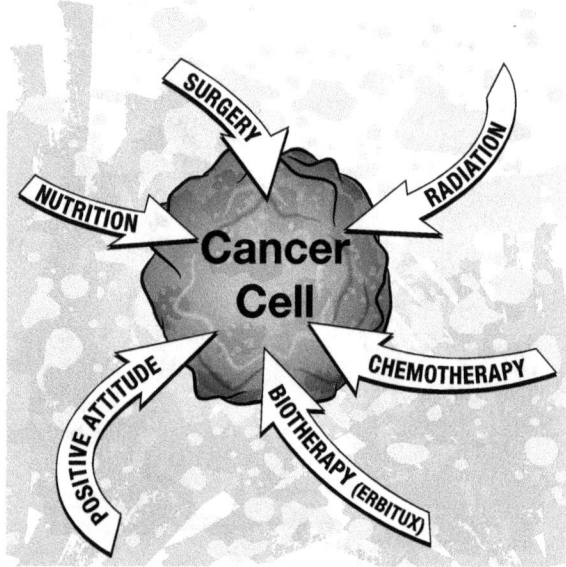

fig. 2.2

Your cancer team will determine the best combination of therapies to attack the cancer cells.

THE SPECIALISTS WHICH COMPRISE THE MULTIDISCIPLINARY TEAM INCLUDE:

- Medical Oncologist (physician who specializes in chemotherapy treatment)
- Otolaryngologist (ENT) or Head and Neck Surgeon (physician who specializes in doing surgery on head and neck cancers)
- Radiation oncologist (physician who specializes in radiation

therapy for cancers)

- Oncology nurse
- Dentist and Oral Surgeon
- Nutritionist
- Speech and swallow therapist
- Audiologist (hearing specialist)
- Stress Management Counselors
- Physical Therapist
- Acupuncturist

fig. 2.3

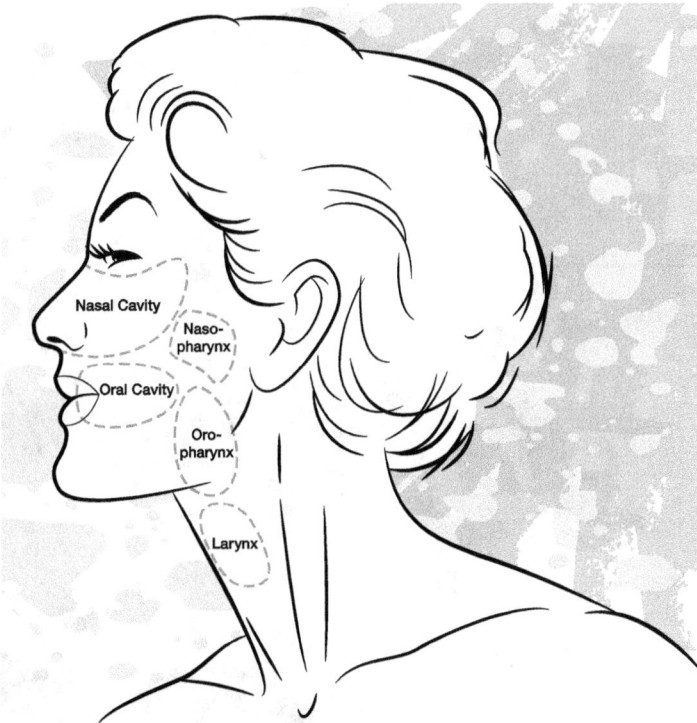

Nasal Cavity

Naso-
pharynx

Oral Cavity

Oro-
pharynx

Larynx

Named anatomic regions in the head and neck

THERE ARE MULTIPLE PLACES THAT CANCERS CAN START IN THE HEAD AND NECK:

- *Nasal Cavity and Nasopharynx:* Area between the eyes and behind the nose. This includes the lining of the walls of this space and the air space.

- *Nasal Sinuses:* These are a group of air sacs within the face. The "Maxillary Sinuses" are spaces found in the cheeks beneath the cheek bones. The "Ethmoid Sinus" is found between the eyebrows, behind the ethmoid bone. The "Spenoid Sinuses" are air filled bones that lie deep near the base of the skull behind the sphenoid bone.

- *Oral Cavity:* This area includes the lips, gums (gingiva), cheeks, tongue, floor of the mouth, hard palate and the retromolar trigone (area inside the angle of the jaws).

- *Oropharynx:* The Oropharynx contains the soft palate (including the uvula, which is the soft tissue that hangs down in the back of the throat), tonsils, base of the tongue (part of the tongue that you cannot see because it is diving down into the throat), and the walls of the throat (Pharynx).

- *Hypopharynx:* This area is the lowest part of the throat before the voice box. It includes the air spaces on either side of the voice box (pyriform sinuses), and the walls of the pharynx at the level of the voice box.

- *Larynx:* This is the voice box and is made up of multiple organs. These organs include the vocal cords (glottis larynx), and tissue above (supraglottic larynx) and below (subglottic larynx).

• *Lymph Nodes:* Lymph nodes are small round oval immune system structures that filter and process foreign debris from things like infections and cancer. They are connected by lymphatic vessels and are throughout the body. When they are fighting cancer or infections, they swell and become larger. This can often be felt or seen on imaging tests like CT scans or MRI scans.

fig. 2.4

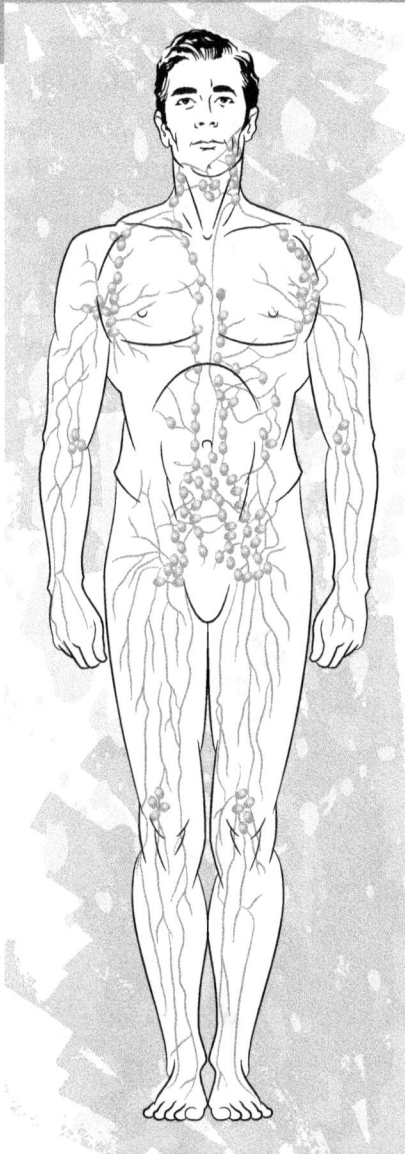

Lymph nodes are small round oval immune system structures that filter and process foreign debris from things like infections and cancer.

As can be seen in fig. 2.2 (pg. 10), this team is a composition of cancer specialists and physicians as well as a support team of other health resources for patients undergoing treatment. For example, Stress Management Counselors are trained counselors who assist patients in dealing with the stress involved with a cancer diagnosis and help to lessen the impact this added stress can have on multiple facets of life.

During the initial time of your diagnosis, your cancer team will meet as a group and will discuss whether surgery is recommended (based on your type of cancer and extensiveness) or if you will undergo non-surgical treatment. It is typical in many situations for surgical treatment to be recommended (particularly if the cancer is on the tongue or in the oral cavity or involving bone). The extensiveness or known spread of the cancer will play a role in determining which treatment will be initially performed and how to sequence individual treatments.

CANCER STAGING

Your cancer stage is determined in general by three assessments.

1. An assessment of how extensive the cancer is at the area of origination (this is given a "T stage" for tumor stage).

2. An evaluation of the nearby lymph node regions is made (this is given a "N stage" for nodal stage).

3. An evaluation of other organs in the body such as the lungs and bones is made to determine if the cancer has spread through the bloodstream to another organ (this is called the "M stage" for metastasis stage).

Your cancer team will give you the T, N, and M stages after they have completed your evaluations prior to treatment and with this information they will discuss the best forms of treatment for your cancer.

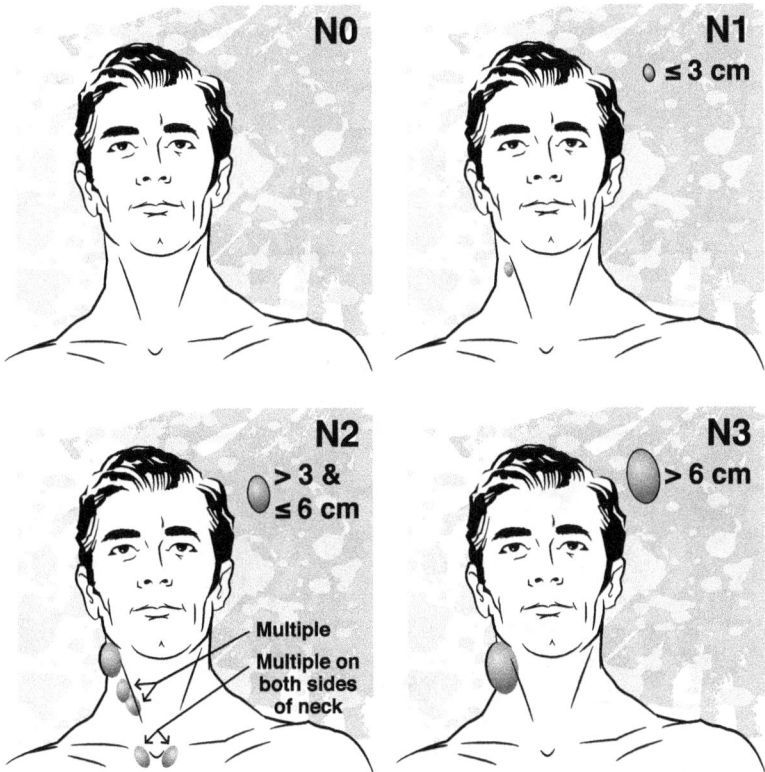

fig. 2.5

This diagram illustrates the different "N stages". The N stage is based on the number of lymph nodes enlarged and their sizes.

PART THREE

Will I Need Surgical Treatment?

HEAD AND NECK SURGERY CONSULTATION: WHAT PATIENTS SHOULD EXPECT

What should patients expect when they are sent to a surgeon for a biopsy?

When patients are scheduled for surgical consultation for a head or neck mass or ulcer, they typically have an appointment with a physician trained in Otolaryngology-Head and Neck Surgery (ENT). The goal of this first office visit is to obtain a thorough history relative to the presenting complaint and to perform a complete head and neck examination.

If an ulcer or mass is found, on examination, to appear abnormal, a biopsy is frequently considered. This can be performed in the office with fine needle aspiration (FNA) and 'punch' or forceps biopsy.

fig. 3.1

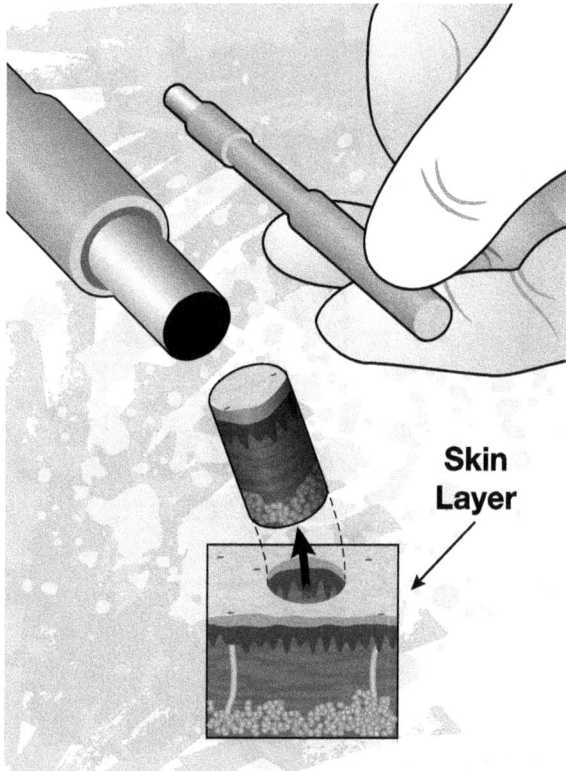

Skin Layer

A "punch biopsy" removes a cylinder of tissue for the pathologist to examine under a microscope.

FINE NEEDLE ASPIRATION

For neck masses, fine needle aspiration (FNA) is common. The process involves the application of a sterilizing solution to the overlying skin, injection of local anesthesia (to create numbness), and multiple (thin needle with syringe) biopsies of the neck mass are obtained in an attempt to obtain tissue for histologic diagnosis. This technique may be performed with or without ultrasound guidance. The process is typically quick, associated with only minor discomfort and requires only a small bandage after the biopsy. The results of the biopsy are frequently available within 1 week and can help guide future care choices and imaging.

PUNCH BIOPSY

For ulcers or lesions of the mouth, nasal cavity or skin, an open biopsy with a technique such as 'punch' biopsy is considered (fig. 3.1). The instrument used for this is a circular knife that isolates a small disc of tissue that can be removed with small tweezers and surgical scissors for pathologic examination. The punch biopsy can be from 2 to 5 mm in diameter and is typically performed after the use of local anesthesia (provides comfort with numbness). Bleeding associated with the biopsy may be controlled with the application of silver nitrate topical chemical cautery or placement of a single stitch. For larger masses with bleeding edges or lesions in the throat or nasal cavity, a biopsy with assistance of forceps that extend the ability of the surgeon to sample deeper tissue (with or without endoscopic guidance, this is by using a small camera that is inserted into the nose or mouth for a better look) can eliminate the need for a surgery.

OPERATIVE BIOPSY

For deeper lesions of the throat, typically around the

larynx (voice box) or esophagus, a short outpatient operative biopsy with general anesthesia and the use of endoscopes (small guided cameras inserted through the nose or mouth) may be required.

The biopsy information is a critical portion of a patient's evaluation and should result in a specific tissue diagnosis. After a specific diagnosis is established, additional imaging (enabling accurate knowledge of if the cancer has spread) and consultation with services such as Radiation Oncology and Hematology Oncology may occur.

What should a patient expect on the day of surgery?

On the day of any surgery, whether performed as an outpatient, or if requiring inpatient hospitalization after the procedure, many of the preoperative considerations remain the same. As a general guideline, the surgeon and anesthesia staff will request that you have nothing to eat or drink for at least 8 hours prior to surgery. If daily medications (such as for blood pressure control) need to be taken on the morning of surgery, a small quantity of water (not coffee or juice) may be used to assist in swallowing these pills. It is always best to check with your surgeon concerning specific preoperative instructions that apply to you in this setting.

If you do not feel well prior to the date of surgery and suspect you may have an upper respiratory infection, contact your surgeon's office immediately for potential re-scheduling of your procedure (your surgeon

NURSE'S NOTE:

Take good care of yourself prior to surgery. Stay away from people with coughs, colds, and fevers. Drink lots of fluids to support your vascular system and kidneys.

would like you to be as healthy as possible for the procedure). If you are a smoker, smoking cessation prior to surgery is in your best interest and will help you with your ability to tolerate anesthesia, postoperative wound healing and your long-term overall health. If you are taking ibuprofen (Motrin, Advil, etc), aspirin or nutritional supplements (such as vitamin E, gingko, ginseng, garlic) discuss this with your surgeon since you will likely be asked to stop taking these medications for at least 2 weeks prior to surgery in an attempt to minimize bleeding during and after the procedure (these are potential blood thinners).

When you arrive on the day of surgery, anticipate that jewelry (including rings and piercings) will typically need to be removed prior to any procedure. In the pre-anesthesia area prior to surgery, you will typically meet with the surgical and anesthesia staff. You should have a full list of all medications (including doses) and allergies available for the staff to review at this time. The name and phone numbers of your family members that should be contacted after surgery should also be reviewed with the staff at this time. Consent for surgery will be reviewed, intravenous lines will be placed and sedation may be initiated.

What should a patient expect after surgery?

The complexity of the surgical procedure and the need for hospitalization afterward will have the biggest impact on the next few days after surgery (postoperative course). For outpatient procedures, you will need to be able to demonstrate an ability to

NURSE'S NOTE:

It is always helpful to carry an updated medical list with you in your purse or wallet for medical visits and in times of an emergency.

tolerate liquids, have adequate pain control and have no significant swelling or bleeding associated with the procedure to be released to go home after the procedure. Prescriptions, if not already provided at your preoperative visit, will be given to you at this time in addition to wound care instructions and the timing of follow-up visits. The final pathological results from a biopsy or procedure can take approximately one week to return, yet in some cases preliminary "frozen section" results (immediate review of the specimen while you are asleep in surgery) may be available on the same day of surgery.

For patients requiring hospitalization after surgery, the goal of care remains similar to the outpatient setting: maintain adequate hydration and nutrition, insure safe breathing, carefully watch wound healing, and provide adequate pain control. If you require a prolonged hospitalization, your physician may request a physical therapy and occupational therapy evaluation and you may be considered a candidate to be transferred to a rehabilitation facility for additional care prior to returning to home.

Your first postoperative follow-up visit with your surgeon will likely review the pathologic results of the procedure, assess the operative site for adequate wound healing (removing sutures or staples) and develop a plan for your next stage in care. If a tracheostomy or feeding tube has been required, additional teaching and care plans will be reviewed with you.

What are some common issues patients should be

aware of after surgery?

Pain is typically addressed while in the hospital with intravenous medications, while oral medications are given typically for pain control at home. Oral medications (like Percocet or Vicodin) are combinations of a narcotic with acetaminophen. Do not take additional acetaminophen (Tylenol) in addition to these medications because this can damage your liver. It is worth noting that all narcotics can aggravate constipation and stool softeners should always be considered (it is recommended to take these for prevention of constipation when on narcotic pain medications).

If wound site experiences significant changes during the first few weeks after surgery (examples are redness, warmth, drainage of fluids, progressive neck swelling, or the onset of bleeding), your physician should be contacted immediately to be made aware of these findings.

Postoperative wound infections are uncommon but can appear days after surgery with increasing pain, smelling, redness, associated fever, and potentially a foul swelling discharge at the operative site. If your wound is not improving with each day of your recovery (relative to pain and the need for care), you may need to be re-evaluated by your physician. It is OK to contact your care team with any questions that you have during this time of healing. They expect you to let them know if you are noticing changes.

For patients undergoing a neck dissection (this is

NURSE'S NOTE:

Remember to take pain medications with food, so that they don't cause an upset stomach.

NURSE'S NOTE:

Some pain medications can be prescribed as a liquid or on a skin patch if you are having trouble swallowing pills.

NURSE'S NOTE:

It is best for male patients to use an electric razor after surgery. The sense of touch in the area may not be the same and the sensitive skin could be easily cut during shaving with a blade or razor.

surgical removal of lymph nodes in the neck), unique symptoms after surgery can develop. The lower portion of the facial nerve (called the marginal mandibular nerve) that provides nerve control to the lower lip may be weak from stretching during the surgery. This can cause a facial asymmetry with smiling and mouth opening. If this is from retraction (stretching) of the nerve during surgery, the nerve should slowly return to function over the next 2-4 months. Shoulder weakness can also be a common result of retraction (stretching) of the spinal accessory nerve and may require physical therapy during recovery. Skin numbness on the same side of a neck dissection is common and often slowly improves over the next 3-6 months after the procedure.

Scar maturation occurs over a period of 6 – 9 months after surgery. During this time, the firm fibrosis (tissue thickening) of the original scar tissue softens, the redness of the incision fades, and the stiff sensation of the affected area loosens. It is for this reason that scar revision surgeries are typically not considered until 6 months after the original surgery.

WHAT IS ENTAILED WITH SOME OF THE COMMON HEAD AND NECK SURGICAL PROCEDURES?

Lymph node biopsy – A lymph node biopsy (requiring an incision and removal of the entire lymph nodes) may be necessary to confirm a diagnosis that a needle biopsy could not. A small, 3-5 cm, incision is created over the area of the enlarged node to allow adequate visualization and removal of the selected lymph node with protection of important surrounding structures. Bleeding is typically minor and placement of a drain is not generally necessary. The incision may be closed with absorbable (does not require removal) or non-absorbable suture (stitches) and these small incisions are usually well healed in about 1 week.

Neck dissection (surgical removal of entire chains of lymph nodes in the neck) – Neck dissection types varies from selective neck dissection (smaller incision and less lymph nodes removed) to modified and radical neck dissections.

1. *Radical neck dissection* involves the removal of all of the lymph nodes (levels I–V, fig. 3.2) on one side of the neck in addition to the internal jugular vein, sternocleidomastoid muscle and the spinal accessory nerve. The aspect of this surgery with the greatest potential for problematic side-effects relates to the removal of the spinal accessory nerve, which can result in a painful shoulder syndrome with short term to permanent limitation of arm movement above the level of the shoulder. The modified radical neck dissection removes all the lymph node levels of the affected neck and preserves some of the sacrificed structures removed with radical neck dissection. Both types of neck dissection are typically used for patients with multiple enlarged lymph nodes involved with tumor.

2. *Selective neck dissection* removes only a selected number of lymph node levels. As an example, the "supraomohyoid neck

dissection" (used when removing lymph nodes in the neck of patients with tongue cancer) removes only lymph node levels I, II and III. Selective neck dissections are used when the risk of lymph node spread of tumor mandates treatment yet limited lymph node involvement is noted on exam. Patients recover far quicker with this style of neck dissection and have less in the way of treatment related side effects. Drains, to collect blood and body fluids from operative site, may be used and will be removed when the amount of drainage decreases in quantity.

Primary cancer resection – When tumors are removed a concept called 'wide local excision' is used. To use an analogy, if a tumor is the size of a dime, a quarter-sized piece of tissue surrounding the tumor (in 3 dimensions) is resected. The goal of surgery is to obtain negative margins if possible, which would indicate complete removal of tumor with a margin of normal tissue surrounding the cancer. The resection may require removal of bone and other functional structures (tongue, motor nerves, etc) if necessary to completely remove the cancerous area. The side effects of surgical resection of the primary tumor depend upon the size of the surgery and the area effected. As an example, a tongue cancer resection will be associated with varying degrees of disturbance in speech and swallowing function. The initial speech and swallowing function after surgery will in most cases improve significantly over time (just as is seen in patients with knee replacement surgery that initially need help with walking before they walk independently).

Tracheostomy – This technique is used in the head and neck cancer patient when there is concern that the cancer is effecting the airway in a dangerous way. Tracheostomy is not a permanent procedure and allows for patients to have a safe airway during care. Removal of the tracheostomy tube (aka decannulation) can occur when the swelling from surgery decreases or when the size of the cancer (as with laryngeal cancer) decreases significantly with treatment (such as chemotherapy, biotherapy, and/or radiation).

fig. 3.2

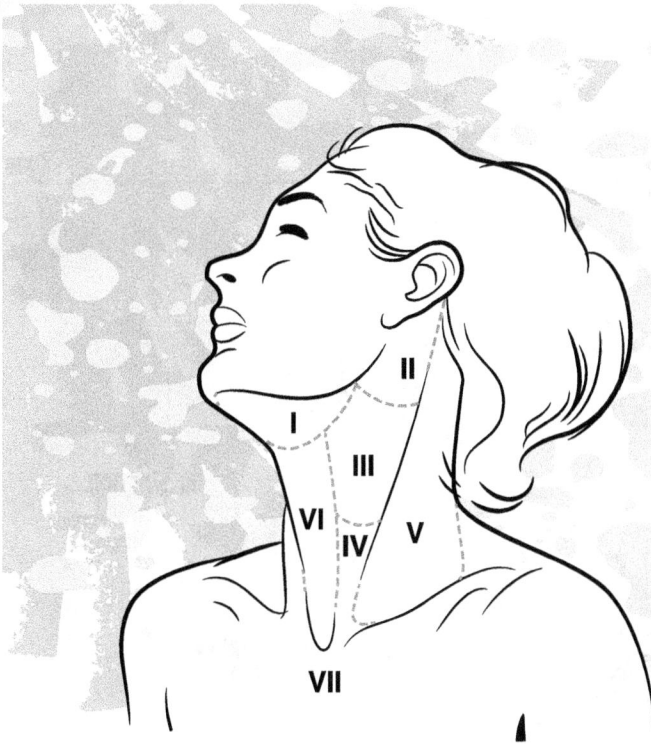

This is an illustration of the common "lymph node levels" in the neck to which cancer can spread. These are the numbers used by radiologists, pathologists, and your treatment team to describe where the cancer is located.

PART FOUR

What Is Radiation Therapy?

RADIATION THERAPY

It's not easy to hear that you or a loved one has cancer. Just the word "CANCER" makes the pulse quicken and brings about fear and uncertainty. Because of this, it's very important to have a team that cares about you to help you through this busy challenging time.

fig. 4.1

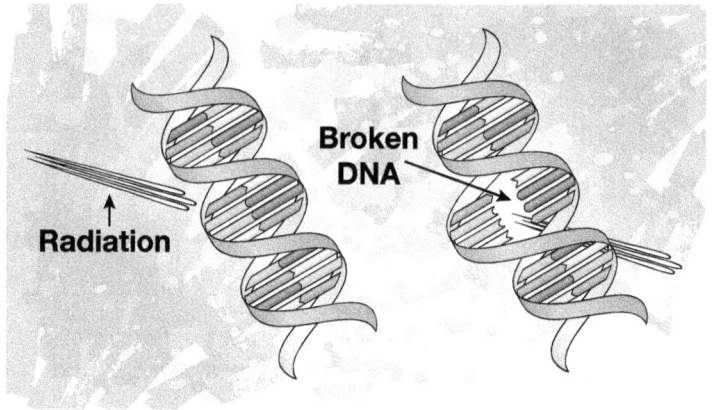

Broken DNA

Radiation

Radiation works by causing breaks in the DNA strands within cancer cells. This leads to cancer cell death.

NURSE'S NOTE:

Radiation Therapists will help you during each day of radiation therapy.

If radiation is part of your cancer treatment, then this can sometimes bring about added fear. You may envision a yellow and black sign warning you "Do Not Enter" and wonder how laying on a bed with beams pointed at you will help get rid of your cancer. For older patients, mental images of past wartimes and radiation drills may increase this fear. You may also know someone that had radiation treatment years ago who got badly burned. I assure you that the technology has come a long way. We have new technologies to very specifically aim the beam at the cancerous areas and protect important parts of your body like your brain, spinal cord, lungs, and heart.

Many advancements have been made over the last decade in radiation therapy and this is a very common standard treatment for head and neck cancer. The types of radiation machines which are used today have the ability to precisely focus radiation on individual areas within the head and neck and protect surrounding critical organs with high precision. Radiation oncologists today can customize therapy for individual patients to make things extremely safe compared to even 10 to 15 years ago. These modern technologies are because of computer advancements as well as advancements in imaging of the body. They plan your treatment with a three dimensional map of your body and can see and target structures just like looking at a GPS localization system of the body.

Prior to performing radiation therapy, a mapping procedure is made of the body. This is called a "Simulation" and involves making an immobilization mold out of a stretchy plastic material which is stretched over the face and upper neck and which hardens at room temperature. This mold or mask verifies and assists in holding your head and neck in the exact same position each day so that the targeting can be exact. Names used to identify modern advancements in targeting include intensity modulated radiation therapy (IMRT), stereotactic body radiation therapy (SBRT), and stereotactic radiosurgery (SRS). The exact type of radiation that would be most beneficial in each circumstance should be, of course, discussed with your individual physician team based on your diagnosis.

When you arrive for radiation treatment, you will be greeted by a radiation nurse or therapist. These folks are specially trained to treat you with radiation for your cancer. The therapist will show you the computer console from which they will be running the machine. They will take a picture of you for their records/chart

NURSE'S NOTE:

Stereotactic radiosurgery is a specialized form of radiation that delivers a highly precise dose of radiation to a small area in a single dose. This is usually done with a head frame ring mounted to the skull with screws.

NURSE'S NOTE:

Many types of special machines have been developed to treat cancer. The most common machine is called a linear accelerator.

and ask you the spelling of your name and your birth date. They will walk with you to the radiation treatment table and help you into the daily specific treatment position. You will likely have a mask (made of soft plastic mesh that they have custom fit for you) placed over your face. The therapist will check several things to make sure everything is accurate and safe before starting the treatment. They won't be able to stay in the room with you, but they will be watching you on a camera from the treatment console. They will also be able to hear you. Some people choose to open their eyes and some keep them closed (either one is safe, so it's whatever is comfortable for you).

fig. 4.2

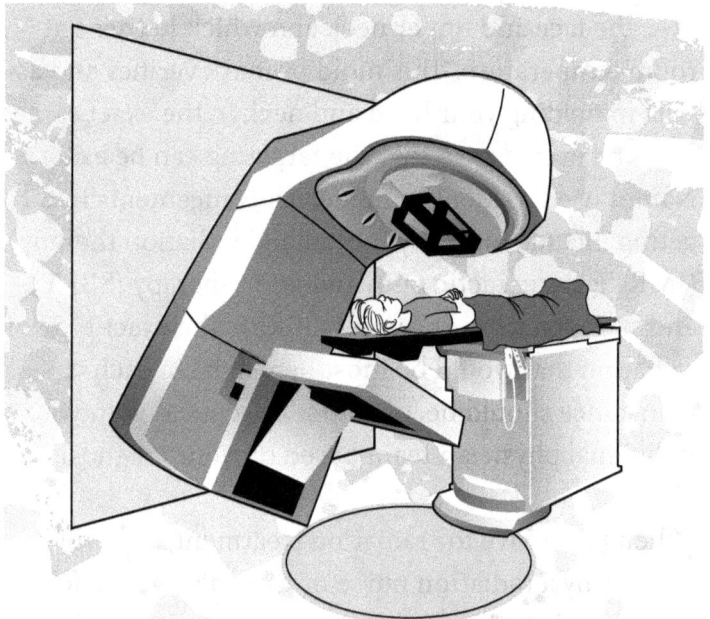

The most common machine used for radiation treatment is called a Linear Accelerator.

When your treatment starts, you will hear some "machine type" clicking and beeping sounds. Patients have related this to buzzing, grates moving, a humming type sound, or a series of clicks. The machine will rotate around you and you will remain in the same position throughout the treatment. Nothing but the mask will touch you during this time. Each treatment is typically very quick lasting between 10 and 15 minutes. These will be five days a week, Monday through Friday, at the same time every day. It is important to make it to every appointment as this will help improve your outcome.

Your nurse will go over skin care the first week of treatment. They will teach you how to take good care of it and help reduce some of the side effects of radiation. They will give you a handout explaining side effects and go over it with you. They will also answer any questions you have and supply you with lotions and creams to start using. Nurses are here to help you get the assistance you need and to assist in providing emotional support during your treatment. Please let your nurse know what she can do for you.

Once a week during your treatment, you will be seen by a radiation doctor. The nurse will also weigh you on a weekly basis. This is very important as you could find it challenging to eat and drink during treatment when swallowing becomes difficult. If your weight loss is worrisome to the doctor or if you are feeling light-headed or dizzy, it could be a sign of dehydration. If this is the case, the doctor may order labs and have you get an IV fluid infusion to help you feel bet-

NURSE'S NOTE:

Wearing a lead apron or shield over the thyroid gland is not recommended during therapeutic radiation treatments because of the energy of the radiation used. These shields would not protect you and could actually make the radiation cause more side effects.

NURSE'S NOTE:

Try not to miss any appointments for radiation therapy. The treatment becomes less effective if days are missed during the treatment weeks.

ter. Pain and nausea medicines can also be given in your IV if needed. We will answer any questions you have at this time and help you manage any side effects that you may be having.

After you are finished with treatment, continue to use your lotions and creams until you come back for your follow up appointment. This will help your skin to continue to heal and provide a barrier for infection. If you have open sore areas on your neck, the nurse may apply a special dressing to help you feel more comfortable and aid in healing. Remember, just because you are done with treatment doesn't mean you are done with our care. You may call at any time with questions or concerns regarding radiation or any other issues. You may be out of our sight, but not out of our thoughts!

SUPPORTIVE CARE

Fortunately for patients undergoing treatment these days, the science of supportive care has advanced in major ways. The biologic causes of symptoms such as nausea, nerve pain, bone pain, poor appetite, and fatigue are being studied. By greater study, improved treatments are already available and additional improvements continue to be made. These improvements allow patients to focus on what matters most: family, friends, work, enjoying hobbies, and thriving in life. At the same time, natural approaches have also improved outcomes by optimizing exercise, diet, meditation, and other alternative forms of therapy.

As part of the initial diagnosis, it is common to discuss and to undergo a **dental evaluation**. Because of the later long-term and permanent effects of radiation on the jaw bone (radiation causes lower blood flow to the jaw bone) as well as the radiation effects on the salivary glands, an increased risk of cavities is very common. It is recommended that all patients undergo a full dental evaluation by their Dentist or Oral Surgeon prior to the radiation being started, so that all dental issues can be repaired up front and future problems can be prevented. As part of this initial evaluation, it is also important for good education to be given to you about fluoride use. Custom fluoride trays can be made by your Dentist for fluoride treatments as well as prescription fluoride toothpaste can be given. After completing head and neck cancer treatment, it is recommended that routine dental visits be done for the rest of your life at four to six-month intervals so that regular cleaning and inspection of your teeth can be performed.

If surgical procedures are needed to the jaw bone or extractions are needed down the road after treatment, some patients require an additional treatment along with dental work, which is called hyperbaric oxygen therapy. This is a procedure which involves daily treatment with high-pressure oxygen therapy which aids in healing of the jaw and surrounding tissues to prevent or to treat a problem called osteo-radio-necrosis (bone death due to poor blood flow and treatment).

Many patients have questions regarding their radiation treatment and this can often be a very challeng-

NURSE'S NOTE:

A full dental evaluation is recommended prior to starting radiation treatments.

NURSE'S NOTE:

Examine your mouth, lips, and tougue daily and let your nurse know if you have mouth or throat pain or are developing sores or a white coating on your tongue.

ing treatment to undergo. It is important to understand that a radiation dose is painless and with each radiation treatment there is no sensation of receiving the treatment. In most cases, the radiation therapy involves a daily treatment of 10 to 15 minute length, five days a week. This treatment is usually for a six to seven week time period. As stated previously, the radiation is painless and there is no sensation of zapping, frying, sizzling, or discomfort. The radiation does have side effects, but these side effects usually happen slowly and over the course of therapy and resolve over the following weeks or months. It is very common for someone who undergoes radiation treatment to experience fatigue, dry mouth, tissue irritation, and a sunburn-like effect on the inside of the throat and mucous membranes of the mouth. This can cause discomfort and sores to form on the surfaces of the tongue, mouth, and throat as well as behind the nose and nasal cavity and can cause short-term and long-term changes to taste, swallowing, and appetite.

NURSE'S NOTE:

The therapists see your skin every day. They will let the nurse know if they are concerned about any areas being treated.

During radiation therapy, there are many things that can be done to improve quality of life. There are multiple types of skin creams that can be utilized to moisturize the skin and to help it to heal in the quickest and most effective way. There are also mouth rinses as well as mixtures of medications which contain lidocaine or other pain medications which can help to numb up the mouth and throat and to improve the ability to swallow and to maintain nutrition. These solutions are commonly prescribed when the sore throat begins along with a mouthwash that can be swished and swallowed and coats the inner surfaces of the throat and esophagus called Carafate. If the skin becomes blistered and peels (desquamation), then other burn creams can be utilized. Some of these burn creams contain antibiotics to reduce the risk of infection.

After the radiation is completed, the majority of the side effects that are experienced during radiation begin to dissipate over the next 10 to 12 weeks. It is recommended that during this time, the patients follow up closely with their physicians so that they can be often monitored and appropriate supportive medications and skin creams can be provided.

One key factor which should be discussed when anyone is diagnosed with head and neck cancer, is the importance of nutrition. In some patients, they are able to maintain their nutrition by swallowing throughout their entire treatment. This is often recommended if possible, as the swallowing muscles can atrophy and develop scar tissues in them if not utilized. In some cases, patients are unable to maintain their nutrition because of the location of the tumor or other health circumstances and a feeding tube may be recommended. A feeding tube is usually recommended to be used on a temporary basis and can become a lifeline for patients during therapy. This feeding tube can be placed by a gastroenterologist or an interventional radiologist through the abdominal wall directly into the stomach or first part of the intestines. Through this tube, medications as well as nutrition can be pumped so that optimal nutrition can be maintained. As previously noted, this can become a

NURSE'S NOTE:

For a dry mouth, try drinking water with dilute lemon extract added (add a cap full of lemon extract to a bottle of water), ginger ale, papaya juice, or rinsing with salt water. The fact is that your mucus will be thinner and more watery if you are better hydrated.

NURSE'S NOTE:

Some patients are more comfortable sleeping in an easy chair or propped up on pillows to aid in swallowing and lesson the chance of choking or gastric reflux.

NURSE'S NOTE:

It is recommended that you avoid high doses of antioxidants during the weeks of radiation treatment because this could possibly protect your cancer from the radiation cell kill.

lifeline for patients and can help to relieve weight loss and fatigue due to malnutrition for many patients. There are many medications that contain antioxidants. It is important to note that antioxidants should be avoided during radiation therapy as the radiation works as an oxidizer; therefore, it is recommended that patients taking supplemental antioxidants discontinue this use until at least 24 hours after the completion of their radiation treatment course.

NURSE'S NOTE:

Please carry a full up-to-date list of mediations you are taking. It is important to include both prescription and non-prescription medications and dietary supplements.

PART FIVE

What Will I Experience During Chemotherapy Or Biotherapy Treatment?

INITIAL MEDICAL ONCOLOGY CONSULTATION FOR HEAD AND NECK CANCER

Patients with head and neck cancer can be treated with surgery, radiation, and chemotherapy depending upon advancement of the cancer (cancer stage) at the

NURSE'S NOTE:

*Medical oncolo-
gists will oversee,
if needed, the
chemotherapy
or biotherapy
portion of your
treatment.*

time of diagnosis. Chemotherapy has been used in combination with radiation for more advanced disease stages, or as a single modality in case of widely disseminated (metastatic) disease. It is of outmost importance for patients to be familiar with the type of chemotherapy that is being used, common side effects and conditions that require a doctor's immediate attention (for example: fever, drug overdose, other very intense signs and symptoms).

What should patients expect during the initial consultation with a medical oncologist?

The diagnosis of head and neck cancer can be quite disturbing to patients and their families. Patients should always try to come for their initial and subsequent visits with member(s) of the family or close friend(s) who they want to share the information about their cancer and therapy. The amount of information that you will learn about the cancer itself and the recommended therapy is quite large and complicated. Having another person to listen and participate in these discussions often has a major impact on your overall understanding of the current situation, and potential problems that you may face during and after therapy.

Discussions about therapy should start with determination of the stage and type of cancer. Imaging studies (CT scans, PET/CT scans, MRI-s) should be reviewed with you (it is good to ask your physicians to review the pictures with you so that you have a better understanding of what organs the cancer has effected). Understanding of the extent of the disease will help you to understand the rational for setting up the appropriate treatment plan. In case of head and neck cancer, the leading rational for chemotherapy or combined chemotherapy with radiotherapy has been preservation of function of the upper digestive and respiratory organs (tongue, larynx, pharynx, etc). Your doctors should review your pathology report with you and discuss what it means. In general, squamous cell carcinoma accounts for more than 90% of all malignant cancers of the head and neck. The other 10% are made up of adenocarcinoma and multiple other more rare disease entities. Once you become familiar with the extent of the disease and appropriate therapy approaches, your Medical Oncologist will discuss the common chemotherapy agents with you.

What should patients know about chemotherapy in general?

Chemotherapy can be given before and during radiation therapy (no evidence supports giving chemotherapy after radiation therapy). Chemotherapy given before radiation or surgery is called induction chemotherapy (this is being further studied and isn't the most common treatment utilized at this time). It usually consists of 2-4 cycles of chemotherapy followed by radiation therapy, surgery, or combined chemotherapy with radiotherapy. This approach is used in select circumstances to reduce the bulk of the cancer before initiation of chemoradiotherapy. However, it is associated with significant toxicity and it is not recommended for all patients with head and neck can-

NURSE'S NOTE:

The type of chemotherapy or biotherapy recommended will be tailored to your situation.

cer. The most common use of chemotherapy is at the same time as radiation therapy to make the radiation work better (called combination chemoradiotherapy). The best studied drugs for this combination therapy are with a standard chemotherapy agent called "Cisplatin" or with a newer biologic therapy called "Erbitux". Both Cisplatin and Erbitux have been recognized on the National Cancer Guidelines (NCCN guidelines) as standard treatment options in combination with radiation for squamous cell carcinomas. Depending upon each person's medical circumstances, other chemotherapy agents can also be utilized and this will be discussed with you by your physician.

fig. 5.1

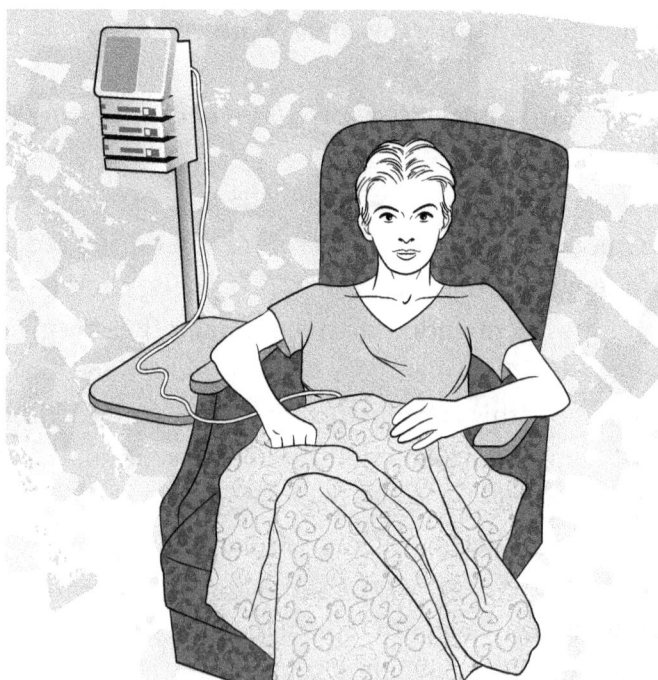

During Chemotherapy, you will be relaxing in a comfortable chair for a couple of hours with the chemotherapy being infused into your bloodstream.

Again stated, the choice of chemotherapy largely depends upon your disease characteristics and overall health. It has been proven that the most important predictor for complications related to chemotherapy is a patient's overall health status (this is termed "performance status"). Good performance status means patient can do all, or almost all, daily activities with minor signs and symptoms of disease. Age alone should not be used as a criterion in selecting appropriate chemotherapy. However, studies have shown no benefit for classical chemotherapy in addition to radiation treatment in patients older than 70 years. Other health issues (heart, kidney or liver diseases) play a major role in determination of appropriate chemotherapy. For example, patients with kidney disease should not be given chemotherapy called Cisplatin since Cisplatin can further compromise kidney function (because of this, they are often given Erbitux due to its safety). In general, patients with poor performance status and with other significant health problems are not good candidates for classical chemotherapy.

Chemotherapy for head and neck cancer is given as intravenous infusion. Commonly, port-a-cath placement is recommended. A Port-a-cath is a small metal or plastic box that has a rubber cover on one side and catheter on the other. It is placed underneath the skin and a catheter is put into a large vein in the chest or arm. Through this "PORT," chemotherapy is delivered directly into a large blood vessel/vein which minimizes the chance of chemotherapy leaking out in the tissue.

On the day of chemotherapy, patients receive anti-nausea and anti-allergic reaction medications followed by chemotherapy. In general, most of the chemotherapy drugs do not cause any problems on the day of infusion. Complications usually start a day or two after the infusion. Allergic reactions are the main exception to this pattern. Allergic reactions most often happen soon after initiation of chemotherapy and include signs and symptoms such as rash, hives, itching, shortness of breath, cough and wheezing, as well as swelling of the lips, tongue or throat (this can happen right away after the chemotherapy has started and you will be monitored for these during your chemotherapy visits). It is very important to discuss a history of allergic reactions to different drugs with your care providers before initiating chemotherapy.

THE MOST COMMON SIDE EFFECTS OF CHEMOTHERAPY GIVEN FOR HEAD AND NECK CANCER ARE:

- Nausea and vomiting
- Pain
- Damage of the inside of the mouth and throat (mucositis)
- Decrease in white blood cells, red blood cells and platelets (lower blood counts)
- Diarrhea
- Hair loss
- Fatigue

- Kidney damage
- Skin rash

Individual chemotherapy drugs have a specific set of common side effects and your doctor will discuss these with you (see the following sections about individual chemotherapy drugs).

fig. 5.2

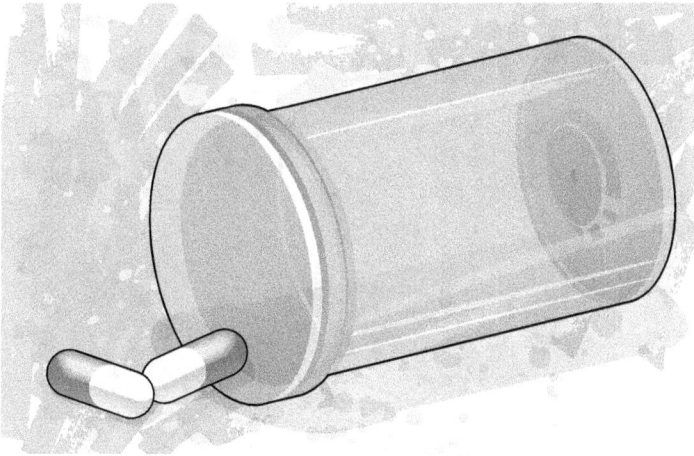

There are many new ways to treat side effects of chemotherapy in this modern day.

Nausea and vomiting. Chemotherapy induced nausea and vomiting (CINV) is one of the most common and feared side effects of chemotherapy. There are three distinct types of CINV:(1) Acute – occurring within one to two hours after chemotherapy and peaking in the first four to six hours; (2) Delayed – occurring more than 24 hours after chemotherapy; (3) Anticipatory CINV – occurring prior to the next treatment.

The objective of anti-nausea therapy is the complete prevention of CINV, and because of modern drugs it can be prevented and treated in the vast majority of people undergoing treatment. This is a big improvement from cancer therapy even 10-15 years ago.

fig. 5.3

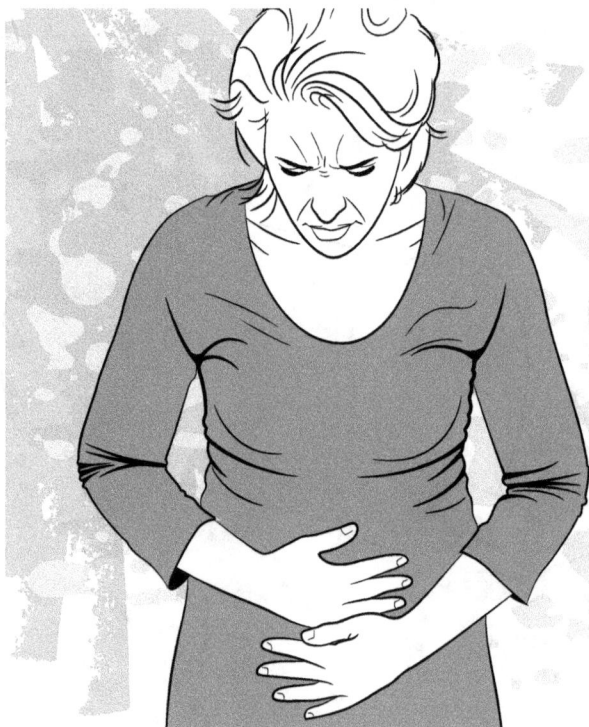

Let your providers know if you are experiencing nausea. With the many new medications available, nausea should not be a big issue for you.

Hair Loss can be a side effect of chemotherapy treatment, but not for all chemotherapy drugs. Of note, radiation treatments can also cause hair loss. Your team will be able to let you know if this will be a side effect of your therapy.

Pain is the result of cancer growing into or pressing on surrounding normal tissues or due to pressure on nerves. Cancer pain is usually treated with opioid drugs (hydrocodone, oxycodone, hydromorphone, codeine, tramadol, etc), or non-steroidal anti-inflammatory drugs (ibuprofen, naproxen, etc). It should be mentioned that opioid drugs have the known potential for abuse and addiction and are given by the prescribing physician in a restricted way for as long as necessary. It is also not recommended to stop the opioid drugs abruptly. Opiod drugs should be tapered down slowly to avoid any severe withdrawal syndromes. Also, short term use and proper tapering prevents the possibility of addiction.

Low blood cell counts (red blood cells, white blood cells and platelets). Almost all classical chemotherapy drugs can have a tendency to decrease blood counts by suppression of the bone marrow. Classical chemotherapy acts against cancer cells by inhibiting their proliferation. Because blood cells also multiply quite fast, chemotherapy will also inhibit blood cell proliferation. Low white blood cell count (neutropenia) is usually treated by giving patients proteins that stimulate white blood cell recovery. Low red blood cells and low platelets are usually treated with red blood cell and platelet transfusions. It is worth mentioning that today's red blood cell and platelet transfusions carry an extremely low risk of HIV and hepatitis infection and they are otherwise quite safe.

NURSE'S NOTE:

Always report side effects to your doctor or nurse immediately, so that they can help support you with medications or other treatments to help you feel more comfortable.

47

Diarrhea. Some of the chemotherapy drugs have tendency to cause diarrhea. Diarrhea is usually treated with drugs that prolong transit time of the bowels, reduce fecal volume and diminish fluid and electrolyte loss.

Skin Rash is a very common side effect of some of the targeted therapies (Erbitux targeted biotherapy). The most common cutaneous change is a "pimple" like (acneiform) rash, most likely present on the face and trunk. It usually begins one week after initiation of the targeted therapy. It is usually treated with topical lotions and steroids, antibiotics, and in extreme cases with oral steroids.

HOW CHEMOTHERAPY WORKS

Chemotherapy is a form of treatment that uses medications to destroy cancer cells. Chemotherapy is usually called "systemic therapy" because these medicines travel throughout the entire body to fight cancer cells anywhere that the blood flows. The goal of chemotherapy is to shrink cancers prior to surgery or radiation therapy, or to add to the effectiveness of radiation. It can also be used to relieve symptoms of cancer such as pain or pressure by cancer on an organ, or to control tumor growth.

It is important to understand how the chemotherapy works in the body. In a normal situation, healthy cells grow by dividing in a uniform and predictable manner. They reproduce and die in a controlled way. As cancer cells grow and multiply in an "out of control" manner, this continued growth causes pressure on other surrounding organs and causes a "tumor" to form. Chemotherapy medicines interfere with this growth. Chemotherapy is particularly effective on cells that divide rapidly. They can also affect normal rapidly dividing cells such as the hair follicles or cells that line the digestive tract. As a result, common side effects from chemotherapy drugs can be hair thinning, diarrhea, nausea, constipation, or mouth sores.

Over the last decade, new designer drugs and targeted agents have been developed. The national guidelines now include use of one of these drugs called Erbitux (cetuximab). The new targeted agent is an artificial antibody which is designed to attach to specific cellular EGFR receptors on the surface of head and neck squamous cell cancers. This drug also has a synergistic effect with radiation therapy (causes the radiation to kill cancer cells more effectively).

There are hundreds of different combinations of chemotherapies. Each medicine, given alone or in combination with other treatments, can cause different side effects, and these side effects will also depend upon your overall health as well as other medical conditions. Chemotherapy is usually given at a cancer center, hospital, or in a doctor's office. The dosage and frequency may vary based upon each person's overall health.

What are chemotherapy/targeted therapies commonly used in head and neck cancer treatment?

Several classical chemotherapies (Cisplatin, carboplatin, paclitaxel, docetaxel, 5-FU) and one targeted therapy agent (Erbitux or Cetuximab) have been used in treatment of head and neck cancer.

Cisplatin is the most commonly used classical chemotherapy drug. Cisplatin harms cancer cells by inhibiting DNA synthesis. It is given as intravenous infusion. Cisplatin causes nausea, vomiting, low blood counts, hair loss, fatigue and occasionally kidney damage and hearing problems. It is usually given with a lot of fluids to prevent kidney damage. It is recommended not to be given if a patient already has kidney damage or hearing problems.

Carboplatin belongs to the same category as Cisplatin. It is commonly given to the patients who are not able to tolerate Cisplatin or other therapies. It is much more tolerable than Cisplatin causing less nausea, vomiting and fatigue. It is usually given in combination with paclitaxel since this combination showed activity comparable to Cisplatin.

Cetuximab (Erbitux) belongs to the category of targeted therapy or biologic therapy. It is an antibody (type of protein) that binds specifically to another protein on the surface of the cancer cells. Binding of cetuximab to the specific surface protein blocks signal that stimulates cancer cells to multiply (fig. 5.4). This interaction causes cancer cell death. It is given as an intravenous infusion. The most common side effects of this treatment is a skin rash. It may also cause allergic reactions, fatigue, dry mouth, dry skin and fatigue.

Docetaxel and *paclitaxel* inhibit cancer cell multiplication by inhibiting DNA and protein synthesis. They are used to treat head and neck cancer under certain circumstances. Paclitaxel is usually used in combination with carboplatin and docetaxel is usually given as induction therapy. Both are given as intravenous infusion. The most common side effects include nausea, vomiting, mouth irritation, low blood counts and possibility of allergic reaction.

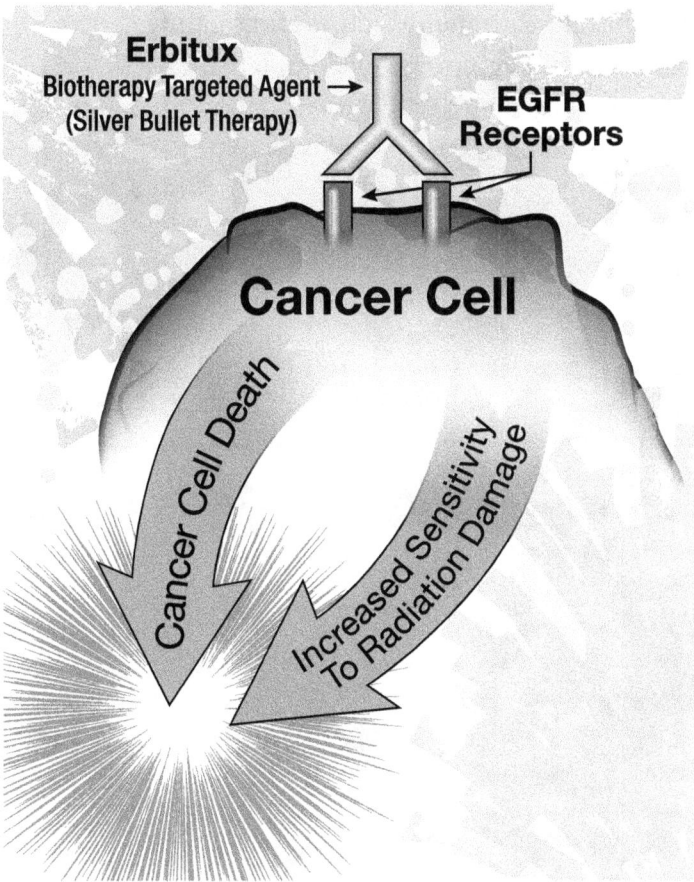

New targeted biotherapies such as Erbitux are "homing devices" programmed to target cancer cells.

COMPLEMENTARY THERAPIES

Many patients inquire today about the use of complementary therapies. Complementary therapies are non-traditional treatment approaches that are used along with traditional treatment. These can be very helpful for many patients and can help in controlling pain symptoms, treating side effects, and improving overall quality of life. These complementary therapies can include massage, homeopathy, meditation, Tai Chi, acupuncture. Of course, it is important that each patient talk with their doctors and treating cancer team before beginning any complementary therapies to verify that it will not interfere with their main forms of therapy.

PART SIX

Focusing On Nutrition

You have been diagnosed with cancer in the head and neck area. You may feel out of control and unsettled right now, but I'm here to tell you how you can be a little bit in control of what may feel like an out of control situation. What you choose to eat can have a strong impact on fighting this cancer. Your immune system is what fights off illnesses and disease. By making the best choices nutritionally, you can maximize your immune system's fighting potential, making you the best cancer fighter you can be. It's all about boosting your immune system, fighting inflammation and decreasing challenges to your immune system so it can focus on the current battle at hand. The information you walk away with today isn't just for here and now, it's for life and long-term health.

fig. 6.1

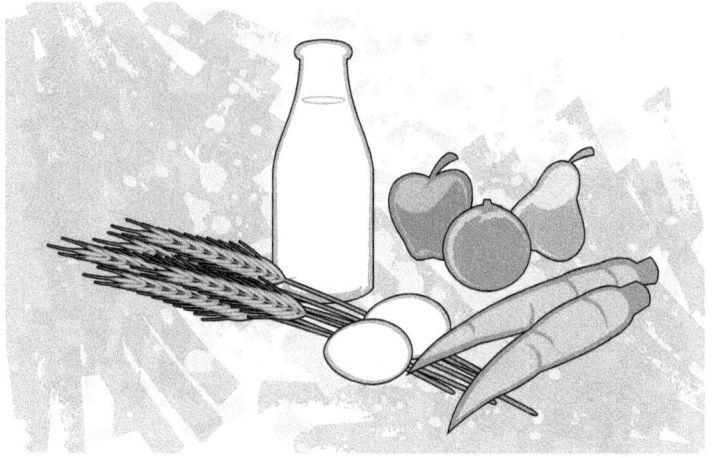

Focusing on nutrition can be the best thing that you can do for yourself during cancer therapy.

IMMUNE BOOSTING NUTRITION

Make every bite count. Well, almost every bite. I like to follow the 80/20 rule. Eighty percent of the time you should make every bite count. Make the best choice for what you decide to fuel your body with. So often we are on the go, or in a hurry, and making unconscious decisions regarding our nutritional intake. Think about it. Is what you are eating doing anything for your body and your fight against cancer? If not, maybe you should think about making some changes in your food selections. That's not to say you can't enjoy those foods that, let's be honest, aren't good for you but they sure taste good and make you feel happy. You can. These are the foods that you have only around 20% of the time. Enjoying birthday celebrations, dessert out with girlfriends, poker night with the guys, whatever it may be, will most likely involve chips, dips and drink choices that you seldom consume. It's OK to enjoy these moments. Make a conscious effort to eat the best you can most of the time, so you can enjoy these special moments and the "not so good" nutrition choices that accompany these occasions without the guilt. It's all part of a healthy eating experience. It's all part of life, as is this current fight you've got on your hands.

Mainly, regarding your diet, the focus should lie on getting back to the basics. Grandma was right! You are what you eat! Having whole foods and less processed foods is where it's at. When buying boxed/convenience foods, select those with less ingredients. Take ice cream for example. It can be a source of protein and calcium, but also has a high content of fat; therefore, only have it occasionally. What I want you to look at, though, is how many ingredients went into the making of it. Buy the ice cream containing only five ingredients or so. Breyers All Natural is a good example of this. I'm not saying eat ice cream all the time, but it is okay sometimes, especially if there are no chemicals/preservatives added to it. This was just an example. In general, focus on eating whole grains, dark and brightly colored fruits and vegetables, plant proteins, lean animal protein sources, fish (especially those high in Omega 3 fatty acids), and other good fats which are listed below. The idea is to balance out carbs and protein at each meal, mini meal or snack. Also by incorporating the good fats into your diet, this will also help in sparing the protein you take in for healing and repair.

WHOLE GRAINS

When choosing whole grain foods, select those that have been the least processed or broken down. Some examples of whole grains include: brown rice, wild rice, whole wheat pasta, quinoa, quinoa pasta, high fiber cereals (hot or cold) containing 5 grams or more fiber per serving, and breads made from whole grain flour, having 3 grams of fiber or more per slice. Whole grain flour being the first ingredient listed. Whole grains have complex carbohydrates in them which are needed by our bodies for energy. They also have protein in them. Quinoa, for example, has 5-8 grams of protein per ½ cup. Give it a try if you haven't already.

PRODUCE

It is recommended that 5 or more servings of fruit and vegetables be consumed each day. This is challenging for a lot of people. What I recommend is to add a fruit or vegetable to every meal, mini meal or snack eaten during the day. Try to eat small meals, every 3 hours or so. At each of these add a serving of produce. Aim for 5 servings a day of dark or brightly colored produce. Some of the best choices include: Broccoli, cauliflower, brussels sprouts, kale and bok choy. These are called cruciferous vegetables and they contain isothiocyanates, specifically Indole-3-Carbinol. This is a cancer fighting compound and should be consumed on a daily basis!

- **Berries of all varieties**
- **Carrots and orange colored produce for the carotenoids**
- **Red grapes for the resveratrol**

- **Green leafies**
- **Tomatoes**

This is a short list of some of the most powerful cancer fighting produce available at grocery stores. It is highly recommended you have your own garden if you can, and grow produce organically. Another thing that should always be mentioned when discussing produce is to wash it in a vinegar and water solution. Wash produce using a solution of 1 Tablespoon vinegar (any kind) in 4 cups of water. This will help to pull off 95-99% of the cancer-causing pesticides used in the farming of the produce. For the thin skinned fruits and hard to wash vegetables, it is better to go organic because it is difficult to completely clean these off. This decreases challenges to your immune system, eliminating one less thing to worry about.

PLANT PROTEINS

Foods of plant origin are high in fiber, vitamins, minerals, antioxidants, beneficial plant compounds, and prebiotic fibers to help support healthy intestinal bacteria balance. Plant based foods are the basis for an anti-inflammatory diet. Beans, legumes, lentils, nuts, seeds, soy foods—these are all sources of protein coming from a plant source. GO FOR IT! Add these to your salads, soups, chili's, or make a bean burger, etc. The list goes on and on.

NURSE'S NOTE:

You may have a nutrition visit prior to starting or during treatment. You will receive a great deal of information. Take a notebook!

ANIMAL PROTEINS

Protein from animal sources is allowed also, but be sure to buy leaner cuts of meat, chicken and other poultry with no skin, and go organic when it comes to purchasing red meat and dairy products containing fat. Buy grass fed cattle because it is higher in Omega-3 fatty acids which are anti-inflammatory. Animal foods, in general, contain higher amounts of Omega-6 fatty acids which are pro-inflammatory so the goal is to decrease intake of animal based foods, while we increase intake of plant based foods and fish, especially those high in Omega-3 fats. (sources listed below) *NOTE: Avoid processed/cured meats due to their nitrite/nitrate content. This is a cancer causing agent used in hams, deli meats, hot dogs, bacon and sausages. Use a nitrate-free product such as Hormel Natural Selections. It can be found in the deli meat section of the grocery store.*

LIST OF PROTEIN FOODS

Beans, legumes, lentils – typical serving size is ¼ cup which equals 7 grams protein. Increase bean intake – try hummus spread, made from garbanzo beans (aka chickpeas).

Nuts, seeds – ¼ cup = 7 grams protein. If nuts and seeds are not tolerated, grind nuts into a spread at your local grocery store. The nut grinders are usually found in the "Health Food" section of the grocery stores by the "All Natural" items.

Milks and spreads/nut butter made from plant foods – almond milk, soy milk, soy yogurt, grind any nut to make a nut butter at your local grocery store.

Fish – especially wild caught salmon, tuna, halibut, mackerel and rainbow trout, for their Omega 3 fatty acid content. Omega 3's, as stated previously, are a natural anti-inflammatory and should be consumed

2-3 times per week. Other fish do not contain high levels of Omega 3's, however, are lean protein sources, with 4 ounces being a serving of fish it provides 28 grams of protein.

Eggs are a high quality protein – each egg has about 5-7 grams of protein. Suggest having 5 eggs a week and unlimited egg whites.

Chicken and turkey – no skin, are lean protein sources. Each ounce has 7 grams protein.

LEAN cuts of red meat –sirloin, ground sirloin for burgers versus ground chuck, and flank steak for fajitas, for example, would be okay for consumption. Also, look for grass-fed cattle as this meat will have more Omega 3's versus the inflammatory Omega 6's. The American Institute of Cancer Research (AICR) recommends limiting intake of red meat, to about 3 servings per week.

Greek yogurt – has about 12-14 grams protein in it and the live cultures (probiotics) will help to normalize gut flora and promote bacteria balance in the intestines.

Low or no-fat dairy – skim milk, 1% milk, low-fat, skim mozzarella, etc. When buying a fat-containing animal product it is recommended to go organic. Look for this statement or something similar on the label, "No hormones or antibiotics were given to this animal or used in the making of this product." Keep in mind when buying fat-containing animal foods: hor-

NURSE'S NOTE:

Good nutrition aids in healing. Make sure to eat a well rounded diet to help support your immune system and heal quicker!

mones, and toxins given to the animal are stored in the fat of the animal. The fattier the animal food, the more likely you are to consume the bad things stored in the fat of the animal. Safer to go organic when it comes to fat-containing animal products. Wise to spend your money on organic meats and dairy products.

GOOD FATS

Lowering dietary intake of Omega-6 fats (mostly animal foods) while raising intake of Omega-3 fats will help to shift the body into "anti-inflammatory" mode. What are good sources of Omega-3's? High Omega-3 foods include wild caught salmon, tuna, halibut, mackerel and rainbow trout. Also, foods of plant origin will have less Omega-6 fats and some Omega-3's like walnuts and flaxseed oil. Extra virgin olive oil, canola oil and coconut oil are examples of good fats as are avocados, nuts and seeds. Daily intake of a ¼–½ of an avocado is recommended.

BALANCE, TIMING, and PLANNING!

Fueling your body consistently all day long, every day, will help you maintain an even keel throughout the day and avoid blood sugar peaks and valleys. By staying on an even keel all day you will provide needed support to your immune system so that it can work at its best potential. Blood sugar stabilization is key. The number one thing I hear from patients is, "I don't eat breakfast." Or, "My whole life I've never eaten breakfast." Now is the time for that to change. Try to consume calories, whether it's eating or drinking, within an hour of waking. You need to wake the body up and let it know that nutrition is on the way. If you're not doing this, it is very likely that your metabolism will slow down.

Another very important thing to remember is that caffeine is an appetite suppressant. I have countless people tell me, "I just drink black coffee all morning and I'm not hungry for anything until about 4:00 in the afternoon." The reason one can go so long without having an appetite is due in part to the caffeine intake as it is suppressing the hunger cue. In actuality, you are slowing down the metabolism. What you need now is a well-oiled machine and to stay revved up to support weight maintenance as well as your immune system. We are addressing weight management and immune-boosting nutrition. To continue boosting the immune system and support your cancer fighting body, I suggest trying to eat every 3 hours, trying never to go longer than 4 hours between intake. This will help to support blood sugar stability all day long and keep you and your immune system energized.

Imagine this: your body is a wood stove. You want to keep the fire burning all day long so you need logs (protein foods) and kindling (carbohydrates) every few hours. Why do this? The answer is simple. If your body doesn't have a consistent source of fuel, it will think "uh-oh, I don't have anything coming in", and begin to work its magic in fueling your body, slowing things down if you will and eventually pulling from energy stores. You have stored energy in your muscles and when not properly nourished you may begin to breakdown muscle. A good way to gauge muscle loss is to look at your arms. Look for atrophy (shrinking muscle mass). Notice if there is any muscle or fat loss. Of course, monitor your weight.

It is okay to lose a little bit of weight but you want to avoid significant weight loss during your cancer treatment. Your radiation team will be following your weight status weekly. The registered dietitian on the team will be alerted if you should experience significant weight loss, change in nutritional status, and/or begin to be more symptomatic. A nutrition consult would be beneficial to address symptoms and give you ways to manage them.

SYMPTOMS

Symptoms often associated with radiation to the head and neck region include: dry mouth, mouth tenderness, sore throat, painful swallowing, difficulty swallowing, and intolerance to foods that are either too hot or too cold. During radiation, the body will naturally send lubrication in the form of a sticky thick mucus-like saliva, as well as send inflammation to the radiation site. Sure the body is trying to heal this area, but it can make it very difficult to swallow when this site is in the head and neck region. To manage the sticky, thick mucus-like saliva, it is best to stay hydrated. Drink water or tea constantly to provide yourself with adequate fluids. This will help to thin out the secretions and make it easier to expectorate (cough up).

NURSE'S NOTE:

Adding a few drops of lemon extract to each bottle or glass of water will help "Exercise" your saliva glands and keep them working well.

Dry Mouth/Tender Mouth:

- Sip water and teas frequently throughout the day to moisten mouth.
- Limit caffeine and alcohol intake as they tend to be a diuretic and pull fluid out of the body.
- Use a non-alchohol containing mouthwash such as Biotene.
- Have water/water bottle with you at all times—take frequent sips.
- Consume moist foods such as stews, casseroles, soups, and fruits.
- Suck on ice chips, popsicles, or make slushies if cold temperature foods are desired and tolerated.
- Use broth, gravies, sauces, yogurt, silken tofu (moist and creamy), warm water, juices, milk or dairy alternatives, and coconut milk to moisten foods.
- Eat soft foods such as yogurt, all natural ice cream, oatmeal, pudding, cream of wheat, malt-o-meal, even cooked vegetables such as cauliflower can be mashed to make "mock mashed potatoes."
- Use olive oil, canola oil, and/or coconut oil to make foods slippery and easier to swallow.
- Avoid crunchy textured foods, tough meats, and raw vegetables.
- Chew xylitol based gum. Xylitol is a sugar-free sweetener and does not promote tooth decay. This is available in most grocery stores down the "health food" or "all natural" sections of the store.

- Use a humidifier in your room at night to keep the air moist.
- Moisten lips frequently with lip balm, Aquafor, cocoa butter or olive oil.

NURSE'S NOTE:

When it comes to gum and mints, sugar free is best. Sugar candies can help bacteria grow in the mouth and may worsen mouth sores or increase thrush growth.

Painful/Difficulty Swallowing:

During radiation treatment, it can become increasingly difficult to eat. The first few weeks you may think, "Oh, OK, I can do this, a little Magic Mouthwash and I can eat." Then it may be something like, "Ouch, it's really hurting to swallow solid foods, I'll stick to liquids or soft foods like yogurt, pudding, ice cream…" This throat pain is only going to get worse.

While we want you to continue attempts at swallowing, this can be done with sips of water and caloric liquids such as juices, popsicles, smoothies, protein shakes or slushies, etc. One simple thing you can do is drink a high calorie nutritional supplement. There are many to choose from and you can even make your own using whey or plant based protein powder. One calorie dense drink I do recommend to gain weight after a big weight loss or to prevent this from happening is Carnation VHC (Very High Calorie). This drink, unlike Ensure or Boost, is not available retail. You can ask at your cancer care facility or you can possibly contact a local home health company on your own and ask them if they carry this formula or something similar.

I suggest you drink this throughout the day at a ¼ cup

dose (equivalent to ¼ can), 4 times per day, refrigerating the formula in between drinks. This will equal one can total per day which is 560 calories. This can help to maintain weight, or at the very least minimize weight loss. ***What we don't want to happen is significant weight loss during cancer therapy.*** Weight loss greatly weakens your nutritional status and your fighting power.

fig. 6.2

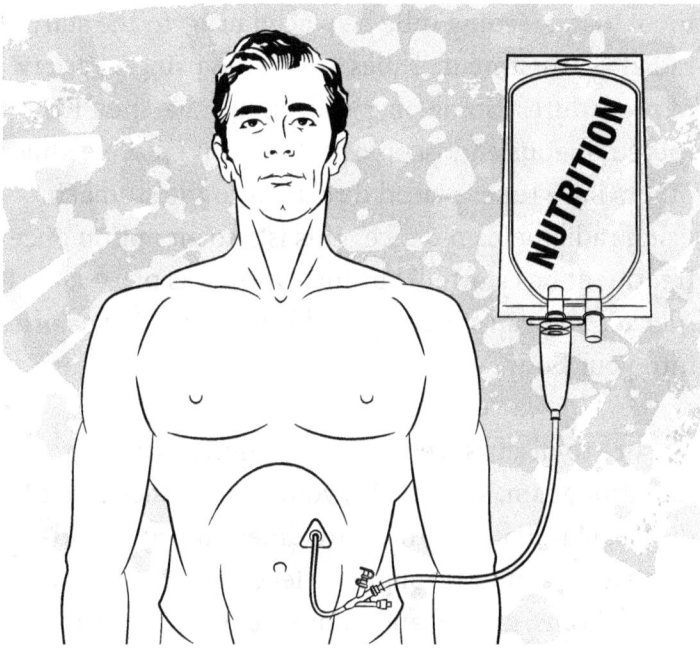

A feeding tube can become a "life-line" for you during radiation treatment if excessive weight loss is a problem.

To prevent weight loss and an impaired nutritional status, the use of a feeding tube is highly recommended for some patients. A feeding tube is a necessary, mostly temporary, means of nourishing your body. It's plain and simple, if you can't swallow your food/liquids you can't meet your nutritional needs. Be proactive and have a feeding tube placed if needed (of course this should be discussed with your health providers to determine if this is best for you).

Once treatment is underway and your esophagus becomes inflamed from therapy, it can potentially be very painful to have the tube placed using an endoscope down your throat. For some patients, it is protocol that a feeding tube be placed prior to the start of radiation treatment. Tubes are placed using a variety of procedures. Some physicians only have the PEG (percutaneous endoscopic gastrostomy) placed while others have tubes placed directly into the stomach using radiologic guidance. This is also an option once treatment has started, but the earlier it is placed, the quicker you can start to get additional needed calories into your body.

Be sure to discuss feeding tube options with your radiation team, specifically, your doctor, registered dietician and nurse. There are different ways to administer feedings through the feeding tube. They are called: bolus, gravity and pump feeds. The only thing that can go in the feeding tube is liquid. There are pre-made formulas like Boost, Ensure, Fibersource, Carnation VHC, or you can make your own mixture if you like.

HIGH IMPACT SNACKS
Consuming foods that provide a power packed punch to oxidants and have a high impact upon every bite

is where it's at! Eating snacks that are high in calories and protein, preferably from a plant source and a source of good fats is the best way to go.

Some examples include:
Trail mix – ¼–½ cup mixture of nuts and dried fruit will give you good fats, carbs, fiber and protein.

Hummus (garbanzo bean spread) – 2 TBSP on whole wheat pita or with 6–10 baby carrots.

A nut butter spread – peanut butter, almond butter, etc. – 2 TBSP on whole grain bread/bagel thin/brown rice crackers, etc.

Protein powder infused smoothie – use whey protein or rice protein. Add to fruit smoothie. Example of ingredients could be: berries, greek yogurt or almond milk, and protein powder. You can add more fruits and veggies to really pack a punch! Do not juice as we want the pulp from the produce because it is loaded with cancer fighting nutrients.

Greek yogurt – has higher concentration of protein. Add a whole grain and or fruit which will work as pre-biotics. Pre-biotics are food for the probiotics that are in the yogurt. The probiotics help to normalize gut flora, therefore, better supporting the immune system.

SUPPLEMENTS
The AICR (American Institute of Cancer Research) has made a recommendation to take minimal supple-

ments while increasing nutrient density of your food intake. We do know from recent research that many of us are deficient in vitamin D. Vitamin D deficiencies are linked with cancer, MS, depression, insomnia, aches/pains, etc. Getting your vitamin D tested is highly recommended and from there it can be determined if vitamin D3 supplementation is necessary.

Fish oil is often recommended because of its anti-inflammatory properties. 1500-3000 mg/day Omega-3's is recommended each day. The Omega-3's are DHA and EPA. Look for the content of these on the back of the supplement bottle. Concentrations vary greatly so be sure to take adequate amounts. If scheduled to have surgery, be sure to tell your surgeon and all physicians involved you are taking fish oil. It is recommended that fish oil be stopped prior to procedures as it thins out the blood.

A multivitamin a day is usually appropriate. Go over contents of it with your registered dietitian and/or doctor.

A fiber supplement such as acacia fiber, is beneficial if you are prone to constipation or extreme cycles of diarrhea then constipation. If you have increased fiber in your diet by incorporating whole grains, fruits and vegetables, supplementation may not be necessary.

The great debate continues on whether to take antioxidant supplementation during treatment or not. Recommendations vary greatly on what is allowed or not allowed during treatment and you will need to discuss this with your oncologists. One thing I tell patients is to listen to your body. You have a mind/body connection and need to listen to it. If you feel confident that something is working for you, then do it. Don't do some supplement just because someone told you about it and it worked for them or because that is what you read on the internet. Of course you will get tons of advice at every turn, but take time to digest it all and figure out what works for you. Rather than focusing on supplementation for added nutrients, it is better to focus on maximizing your nutrient intake through food. You can go to *www.ORACvalues.com*. ORAC stands for oxygen radical absorbance capacity, which is the antioxidant power of foods. *ORACvalues.com* is a comprehensive database of foods and their antioxidant levels. Some things high in ORAC are: parsley, blueberries and cinnamon. Check out the website to see what others are high in ORAC values!

NOTE: Always discuss all meds, natural supplements, vitamins and minerals with your doctor to assure nothing is compromising your treatment.

RECOMMENDED BOOKS

Eating Well Through Cancer – distributed by Merck

The Cancer Lifeline Cookbook – by Kimberly Mathai MS, RD, with Ginny Smith

The Cancer-Fighting Kitchen and One Bite at a Time – by Rebecca Katz

In the above-mentioned books you will find whole-foods based recipes and wonderfully helpful nutrition information.

I would like to address the world of online information. You will see many things on the computer. "Googling" has become a way of life but be careful in what sites you go to. There is one theory found online that gets brought up the most. It is the theory that "sugar feeds cancer." I want you to remember one thing: anything growing inside of us will be fueled by what we are fueled by. Our main energy source is glucose. This is sugar. As stated before, follow the 80/20 rule of thumb with regards to diet and nutrition. Most definitely do not avoid fruits and whole grains in hopes of depriving your body of sugar or in hopes of starving the tumor. Keep the focus on balance of carbohydrates, proteins, and good fats. Eat whole grains, bright or dark colored produce, plant proteins, lean or lower fat animal proteins, and good fats.

RECOMMENDED WEBSITES

There are numerous websites to view. So much so it can be overwhelming. Below is a list of credible websites.

www.caring4cancer.com/go/cancer/nutrition – the side effects management section is written by a registered dietitian.

www.cancer.org

www.cancerrd.com

http://oralcancerfoundation.org

www.cancer.gov/cancertopics/wyntk/oral

www.nlm.nih.gov/medlineplus/oralcancer.html

www.aicr.org/site/PageServer

www.mypyramidtracker.gov/planner/

www.oralcancerfoundation.org/dental/xerostomia.htm – information on dry mouth.

www.foodnews.org – for the Dirty Dozen annual report on produce.

www.consumerlabs.com – to review your supplement. See if it passed quality testing.

www.ORACvalues.com – to review antioxidant levels of foods.

www.livestrong.org

www.asha.org/public/speech/disorders/SwallowingProbs.htm – American Speech Language and Hearing Institute.

PART SEVEN

Returning To Normal Life

Often, we hear patients state that the initial period after their cancer therapy has finished can be emotionally very difficult. Because they have been focusing all energy and thoughts on fighting cancer and so much time has been occupied by visits with care providers and treatments, it is often hard to return to normal life and to normal activities.

After treatment you will continue to see your cancer team every few months for checkups. Be sure to be prepared for these visits.
- Be truthful about your symptoms and how you are feeling
- Bring your medication list to the appointment
- Make a list of questions that have been on your mind
- Take notes at the appointment
- It is OK to ask your health provider if you may use a tape recorder during the appointment for later review
- Ask a family member or friend to go with you to lend a second pair of ears and to add more questions to the discussion

We recommend that you have a discussion with your care team about plans for the frequency at which you will be examined by your doctors in the future, as well as the future frequency of imaging studies (CT, MRI, or PET scans). It is also important for patients with teeth to undergo routine follow up dental visits for cleaning at four month intervals. Many patients also benefit from undergoing physical therapy for neck and jaw range of motion and stretching exercises. One of the long-term side effects of radiation is fibrosis and thickening of the skin and reduced range of motion of the neck and jaw, which can be helped effectively with physical therapy. Radiation and chemotherapy can also have effects on the inner ear and in some cases hearing aids are needed to improve hearing in the long run.

Dealing with stressful periods of time after cancer treatment, such as awaiting results of scans and blood tests, can lead very frequently to anxiety and depression. These are very common and your health care providers can assist in referrals to counselors who deal frequently with these common symptoms, and in some cases prescription medications can be utilized to ease anxiety and depression. Often times, patients can greatly improve their quality of life by developing positive coping techniques.

WAYS OF COPING

- *Express your emotions*: Many people experience fear, anger, or sadness. Find someone comfortable to talk with such as a friend, family member, or keep a private journal.
- *Learn more about your diagnosis*: Knowledge is power. Many people find that the more they learn about their diagnosis, the less they worry about the future.
- *Work on a Positive Attitude*: Research has shown that people heal better, have better immune systems, and have better treatment outcomes when they can maintain a positive attitude and cope in a positive way with difficult news.
- *Exercise*: Start with small steps and ask your health care providers for advice on what types of exercise will be safe for you and best for recovery. Physical therapy can also often play a role in helping to set realistic goals for physical achievement.
- *Treat yourself to something nice*: You are a cancer fighter and

deserve to reward yourself every day. Do something you enjoy, meet with a friend, watch a favorite movie, or listen to your favorite music. Whatever it is, focus on finding time for yourself so that life is more relaxing and enjoyable.

Depending upon the aggressiveness of treatment and overall health following treatment, many patients set the goal to return to work. It is recommended that this be discussed with your cancer physician team. If full time work cannot be started right away, just starting part time work or easing back into work can be beneficial to quality of life as well as help to ease the financial burden in many patients. Returning to work also helps to "take your mind off of the cancer."

Chronic pain can be an issue for some patients, and this is an issue that also should be discussed individually with your cancer team. In most cases, pain dissipates over a few months after treatment. In chronic situations, a referral to a pain specialist can be beneficial for many patients and, of course, close follow up with your care providers is important due to the side effects of pain medications. In some cases, other complementary specialties, such as acupuncture and chiropractics, can be beneficial for pain syndromes.

It is also important for anyone who has undergone radiation to the head and neck area to be tested periodically in the future for hypothyroidism, as the radiation can have long-term effects on thyroid function. If your thyroid function is found to be low on the blood test, you will be given a medication to make up for the missing thyroid hormone. This medication is very easy to use and very safe for the majority of patients.

Due to surgical and radiation side effects, the ability to swallow can also be impacted negatively. Specialists who are trained in speech and swallow therapy can be extremely beneficial in teaching techniques for improving swallowing function and improving speech for patients with these concerns. In some patients with cancers of the larynx, the voice box is removed surgically. There are also numerous devices available to aid in speech and swallowing for these patients and it is recommended that they work carefully with speech and swallow therapists to optimize their treatment and quality of life.

Where can I find out more information about Head and Neck Cancer?

American Cancer Society
 (800) ACS-2345
www.cancer.org

Cancer Survivors Network
(800) ACS-2345

CancerCare, Inc.
 (800) 813-HOPE
www.cancercare.org

Cancer Fund of America
(865) 938-5284
www.cfoa.org
Cancer Information Service (CIS)
(800) 4-Cancer
www.cancer.gov

National Coalition for Cancer Survivorship
(877) NCCS-YES

National Comprehensive Cancer Network (NCCN)
(888) 909-NCCN

WEBMD
www.webmd.com

PART EIGHT

Your Cancer Journal

YOUR WORKBOOK TO
COLLECT INFORMATION

Date of my diagnosis with cancer?_____

What type of cancer do I have? _____

Where did it start?_____

Has it spread to any other areas?_____

Where has it spread?_____

What is my cancer stage?_____

T_____N_____M_____

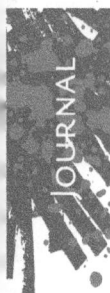

What are my current medications and doses?

1. _____
2. _____
3. _____
4. _____

I am allergic to these medications:

1. _____
2. _____
3. _____

What treatment have my health care providers recommended?

Surgery? _____

Radiation? _____
                    (Type and for how long)

Chemotherapy? _____
                    (Type and for how long)

Who are the care providers on my team? (Phone #)

1. _____
2. _____
3. _____
4. _____
5. _____

Record questions to be asked:

_____

_____

_____

_____

_____

_____

_____

_____

_____

_____

_____

_____

_____

_____

_____

_____

_____

_____

_____

_____

_____

_____

_____

_____

_____

_____

_____

_____

_____

_____

_____

JOURNAL

Notes and drawings:

_____

_____

_____

_____

_____

_____

_____

_____

_____

_____

_____

_____

_____

_____

_____

_____

_____

_____

_____

_____

_____

_____

_____

_____

_____

_____

_____

Record dates and times of new symptoms for your records:

New Symptoms	Date And Time	Severity (1-10)

JOURNAL

Common Cancer Terms

Adjuvant therapy: Treatment used after the main treatment (i.e., after radiation or surgery). As an example, chemotherapy or radiation may be given after surgery to increase the chance of cure.

Base of Tongue: The part of the tongue you can't see that extends down the back of the throat.

Benign tumor: An abnormal growth of cells that is NOT cancer and forms an abnormal lump.

Biopsy: A procedure in which a small piece of tissue is taken for examination by a pathologist to see if cancer is present or not.

Buccal mucosa: The soft lining on the inside of the cheeks.

Cancer: A term used when cells with damaged or abnormal DNA start to grow out of control.

Chemotherapy: Medicine usually given by an IV to stop cancer cells from dividing and spreading.

Computerized Axial Tomography: Otherwise known as a CT scan. This is a picture taken to evaluate the anatomy of the head and neck in three dimensions.

Deoxyribonucleic Acid: Otherwise known as DNA. This is something found in every cell of the body. It is what programs a cell to do specific functions.

Ethmoid sinus: An air space found between the eyebrows and below the bone.

Feeding tube: A flexible tube placed in the stomach through which nutrition can be given.

Gastro esophageal Reflux Disease (GERD): A condition in which stomach acid moves up into the esophagus and causes a burning sensation.

Grade: Term that helps describe the aggressiveness of tumor cells.

Hard palate: Roof of the mouth.

Histology: A description of the cancer cells which can distinguish what part of the body the cells originated from.

Hypopharynx: The lowest part of the throat above the larynx that helps to keep food and fluids from entering the lungs.

Intensity Modulated Radiation Therapy: Also known as IMRT. A complex type of radiation therapy where many beams are used. It spares surrounding normal tissues and treats the cancer with more precision.

Laryngectomy: The term used for surgically removing the voice box or larynx.

Larynx: The voice box (contains your vocal cords).

Localized cancer: Cancer that has not spread to another part of the body.

Leukoplakia: A whitish patch inside the mouth.

Lymph nodes: Bean shaped structures that are the "filter" of the body. The fluid that passes through them is called lymph fluid and filters unwanted materials like cancer cells, bacteria, and viruses.

Malignant: A tumor that is cancer.

Maxillary sinuses: Air spaces behind the cheeks and above the jaw.

Metastasis: The spread of cancer cells to other parts of the body such as the lungs or bones.

Nasopharynx: The air pocket between the eyes and behind the nose.

Neck dissection: Surgery of the neck that removes lymph nodes to check for spread of cancer.

Neoadjuvant therapy: Chemotherapy or radiation that is given before surgery (or radiation) to help shrink the tumor.

Oropharynx: Area made up of the soft palate, uvula, tonsils, base of the tongue, and the walls of the pharynx.

Osteoradionecrosis: Damage to the bone caused by radiation effecting blood flow to the bone.

Otolaryngologist: A doctor that specializes in ear, nose, and throat (ENT).

Palliative treatment: Treatment that helps relieve the symptoms of cancer, such as pain, but does not cure the disease.

Pathologist: A doctor trained to recognize tumor cells as benign or cancerous.

Pharynx: Area of the throat.

Positron Emission Tomography: Also known as a PET scan. This test is used to look at cell metabolism to recognize areas in the body where the cancer may be hiding.

Pyriform sinuses: The air space on either side of the larynx (or voice box).

Radiation therapy: Invisible high energy beams that can shrink or kill cancer cells.

Recurrence: When cancer comes back after treatment.

Remission: Partial or complete disappearance of the signs and symptoms of cancer. This is not necessarily a cure.

Risk factors: Environmental and genetic factors that increase our chance of getting cancer.

Side effects: Unwanted effects of treatment such as hair loss, burns or rash on the skin, sore throat, etc.

Simulation: Mapping session where radiation is planned. If the doctor will be using a mask for your treatment, this is the time it will be custom fit for your face.

Soft palate: Back area that connects to the roof of the mouth and makes up the soft part (this is where the uvula hangs from).

Sphenoid sinuses: Air spaces behind the sphenoid bone.

Staging: Tests that help to determine if the cancer has spread to lymph nodes or other organs.

Tonsils: Soft tissue on both sides of the throat. Tonsils are part of the lymphatic system.

Tumor: A new growth of tissue which forms a lump on or inside the body that may or may not be cancerous.

Uvula: The soft piece of tissue that hangs down in the back of the throat.

About The Authors

Danko Martincic, MD: Dr. Martincic was born and raised in his native Croatia. He graduated as a Faculty of Medicine in Zagreb (Croatia) in 1988, and subsequently moved to the United States in 1991 to pursue fellowship in molecular biology at the University of Southern California. He moved to the Vanderbilt University in 1994 and spent the next six years as a research instructor and associate professor in the Division of Pediatric Hematology/Oncology. His interests were mainly in developing methodology for point mutation detection and the study of mechanisms of resistance to chemotherapy agents. He subsequently completed residency in internal medicine and a fellowship in hematology/oncology at Vanderbilt University. He moved to Spokane to join Cancer Care Northwest in 2006.

Richard O. Wein, MD, FACS: Dr. Wein performed his residency in Otolaryngology-Head & Neck Surgery at the University of Rochester Medical Center in Rochester, NY. He subsequently completed fellowship in Head & Neck Surgical Oncology and Microvascular Reconstruction at the University of Pennsylvania Health System in Philadelphia, PA. He is currently an Associate Professor and Residency Program Director in the Department of Otolaryngology-Head & Neck Surgery at Tufts Medical Center in Boston, MA. His practice and research interests focus on the multidisciplinary management of head and neck cancer and the surgical treatment of thyroid, skin and salivary neoplasms.

Heather Gabbert, MS, RD, LD: Heather attended Southern Illinois University at Carbondale and graduated with her Master's Degree in Dietetics in 1995.

She has been a Registered Dietitian (RD) since and has lived in different areas of the country throughout the years, in each place, gaining valuable experience in the field of dietetics. She has worked with cancer patients since 1998 when she began working at Cancer Treatment Centers of America. Heather moved to Spokane, Washington, from Chicago, Illinois, in 2007 where she worked as an RD for LifeCare Solutions and then CancerCare Northwest. She will be employed by Cancer Treatment Centers of America once again as Nutrition Manager after having been employed at Cancer Care Northwest for 3 wonderful years as oncology dietitian.

Heather is a member of Academy of Nutrition and Dietetics (AND), Washington State Academy of Nutrition and Dietetics (WSAND), and Greater Spokane Dietetics Association (GSDA). She served for two years as Media Representative and board member for WSAND and GSDA. Heather has authored a book, articles and has blogged for StepUpSpokane, highlighting nutrition and wellness. She is a member of AND's DPG groups: Oncology, Business Communications and Entrepreneurs, and Sports, Cardio and Wellness Nutrition (SCAN) group.

Kathy Beach, RN: Kathy graduated with her RN degree in 1993. She decided to get a degree in nursing after her mother was diagnosed with breast cancer. She spent sixteen years in hospital nursing where she worked on a wide range of units from Medical Oncology to Outpatient Surgery. For the past 4 years, she has focused her energy in oncology and radiation oncology with Cancer Care Northwest in Spokane, WA. She loves her work and finds the patients she cares for and their families to be extremely inspiring.

Christopher M. Lee, MD: Dr. Lee graduated cum laude in Biochemistry from Brigham Young University in 1997 which included a summer research fellowship at Harvard University and Brigham and Women's Hospital. He subsequently attended Saint Louis University School of Medicine where he received his M.D. with Distinction in Research degree. He completed four additional years of specialty training in Radiation Oncology at the Huntsman Cancer Hospital and University of Utah Medical Center during which he was given multiple national awards. Dr. Lee has actively pursued both basic science and clinical research throughout his career. He continues to be a proliferative author of scientific papers and regularly gives presentations on radiotherapy technique and the use of targeted radiation in the care of patients with head and neck (throat), brain, breast, gynecologic, and prostate malignancies.